# F\*CKING DEAL
# WITH IT

# For Mom, Dad & Mister

Printed in South Korea

SASQUATCH BOOKS with colophon is a registered trademark
of Penguin Random House LLC.

28 27 26 25 24                    9 8 7 6 5 4 3 2 1

Editor: Sharyn Rosart, Jill Saginario
Production editor: Isabella Hardie
Designer: Tony Ong

ISBN: 978-1-63217-479-6

Sasquatch Books
1325 Fourth Avenue, Suite 1025
Seattle, WA 98101

SasquatchBooks.com

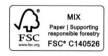

# F*CKING DEAL WITH IT

A Journal for Practicing Acceptance and
Getting the Hell on with Your Life

## SASQUATCH BOOKS
### SEATTLE

# Contents

**91**  PART THREE:

# F*cking Deal with It!

**117**  PART FOUR:

# The Best Is Yet to Come, Baby!

## INTRODUCTION:
# How ACT Saved My AS$

When I got diagnosed with depression in 2018, my first instinct was to "cure" myself. In addition to traditional CBT therapy, I overwhelmed my life with herbs, acupuncture, kickboxing, 7 a.m. pilates, sound baths, tarot cards, crystals, witch candles, vegan donuts, spending money on shoes, calling old friends, making new ones, throwing myself into work, paying off my shoe credit card, putting my bare feet in the grass, making boundaries, cutting my own bangs, falling asleep to ASMR videos of a British woman whispering positive affirmations . . . None of it worked.

Not because anything I tried was inherently *wrong*. In fact, some of it made me feel a lot better! I love tarot cards and acupuncture now.

But the more time I dedicated to curing my depression, the more depressed I felt. It reminded me of that phenomenon where once you notice a clock ticking, you can't unhear it. Your day flips from quiet and peaceful to the never-ending, skull-grating *tick, tick, tick. OKAY I FREAKING GET IT TICK I AM GOING TO JUMP OUT OF MY SKIN.* Enter acceptance and commitment therapy, or ACT.

When I first poked around the concept of ACT, I assumed the acceptance part meant "giving up." As in: "Welp. I have been diagnosed with depression. Better just give up trying to be happy and accept my new role as a Sad Person." However, after studying Steven C. Hayes's thoughtfully crafted ACT workbook, *Get Out of Your Mind and Into Your Life*, I started to see the light. Acceptance absolutely does not mean giving up. Yes, I needed to accept that I will live with depression for my whole life, but it's up to me to decide what living looks like. It's less about trying to get out of the ocean and more about swimming with the tide (hope you like metaphors because that's the first of about eight hundred in this book).

And happy? Pffft. F*ck happiness. Being human means we're capable of experiencing EVERY. SINGLE. EMOTION. All of them! The whole boxed set! Focusing on happiness alone robs you of a full life. It's impossible and, honestly, boring. So, where should we put our focus? Well, that's where the C in ACT comes in. The C is for "cookies," and we gotta focus on cookies as much as we possibly can. Sorry, I'm kidding. C stands for "commitment." We need to decide what we commit our time to (so actually, I guess you could pick cookies if you felt really strongly about it). Steve (can I call you Steve, Steven C. Hayes?) refers to these commitments as "values," but I've also heard this similar concept called "purpose," "calling," and "intention." We'll get into all that mumbo jumbo in Part Four, so get pumped. First, I want to make something clear: this book is not going to magically bring you happiness.

But holy heck, I hope it brings you peace.

Don't give up!

Lots of love,

**Christina**
Sit-Down Comedian,
Professional Depressed Person

# How to Use
# This Workbook

- These exercises are meant to be done in order, but if you get stuck on one, by all means skip it. Tear it out. Throw it into the river. Repurpose it for a cute Etsy product.
- I recommend keeping this workbook in an area where you usually find yourself mindlessly scrolling on your phone, like in the glove compartment of your car or on a cute shelf next to your toilet. You're more likely to make time for it!
- If you're in therapy, talk about these exercises with your therapist. I am NOT a healthcare professional; I am just a girl with depression, anxiety, and a trauma-induced sense of humor.
- And if you're not in therapy? Consider starting the journey. It can be intimidating, but I know you can do it. There are some resources in the back of this book.
- This workbook works best when you use sparkly gel pens. It just does.

# Your First Assignment

Fill out this contract. You can ask a lawyer to look it over for you if you want.

I, _____ , (your name) promise to be
as kind as possible to _____(your
name again) while filling out this workbook. Even
though lots of judgmental thoughts might bubble up,
I will try my best not to give those thoughts power.
Instead, I'll focus on the FACT that I'm a smart,
capable, sensitive li'l human bean taking steps to
make my life better. I won't be mean to my brain
because I love my brain, even with all its faults.
Kind of the same way I love a puppy. Like, yeah,
sometimes my brain metaphorically poops in my shoes,
but I still love it to bits. I understand that this
contract is legally binding* and will sign using
my favorite pen. I will also avoid speaking in the
third person in the future.

Love,

X_____
AUTOGRAPH HERE

*Just kidding. I didn't go to law school. I didn't even google "contract" before writing this.
Please don't sue me.

# PART ONE:

# Why the F*ck Am I So Miserable?!

Let's play detective! Grab your magnifying glass, because it's time to solve the mystery of WHY DOES LIFE SUCK ~~SO MUCH~~ A NORMAL AMOUNT?

Life is pain, Highness. Anyone who tells you differently is selling something.

**—WESTLEY**, *The Princess Bride*

# ICEBERG, DEAD AHEAD

*Of course I talk to myself, because sometimes I need expert advice.*

**—BUGS BUNNY**

You know those days when one little-bitty inconvenience seems to rip open the time-space continuum, causing you to totally break down? Relatable!

It's not really about the itty-bitty inconvenience, though, is it? Our worries, even ones we've carried with us since frickin' childhood, are all connected. So, while on the outside we're upset about running late, our worry goes way deeper, like the underside of a freaking iceberg:

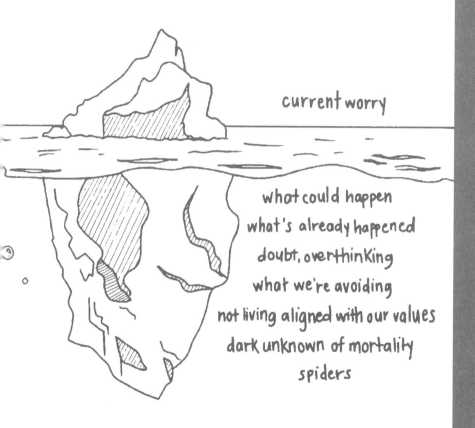

current worry

what could happen
what's already happened
doubt, overthinking
what we're avoiding
not living aligned with our values
dark unknown of mortality
spiders

One of the main goals of the workbook is understanding ✦ acceptance. ✦ Acceptance doesn't mean that when you notice an iceberg in your path, you jump off your boat. Nor does it mean you should hit the throttle, hoping the force of the collision reduces the iceberg to a big ocean slushy. Acceptance means working *with* the iceberg, finding a path around it. The journey might take a little longer than expected, but the point is that you continue the journey!

If we are going to steer our boats around icebergs, we need to be able to recognize them. So here's your first exercise: What's under the surface of your current worry?

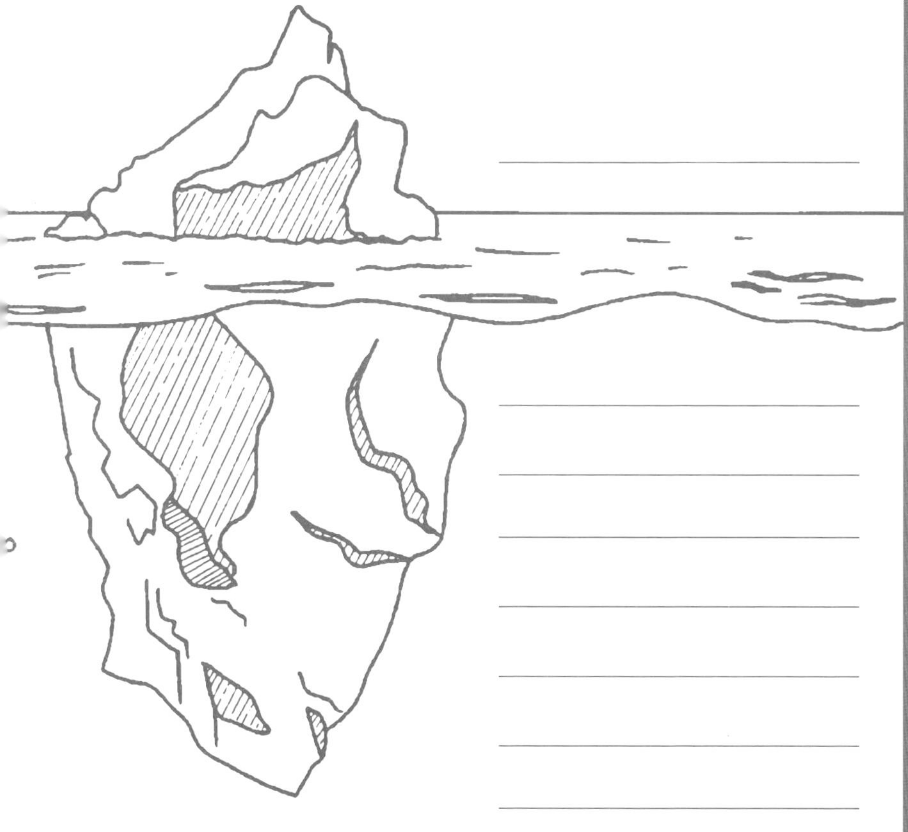

# THE WORST FORTUNE TELLER EVER

One of the best ways to make yourself anxious as hell is believing that you can predict the future. Fortunately, I have very good news for you: your brain's crystal ball is broken. In fact, it never worked, not even a little bit. Instead of trying to return it to Spencer's (we've lost the gift receipt; it's too late), let's examine some times we trusted that defective crystal ball a little too much.

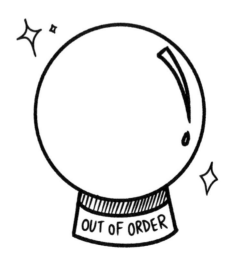

What are some times your anxiety felt like a premonition?

What really happened (*instead* of your brain's *That's So Raven* catastrophic vision)?

See? No offense, but your brain isn't psychic! You just have a powerful imagination. Brain, you're fired!

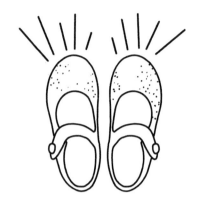

# THROW THOSE RUBY SLIPPERS AWAY

Remember Dorothy? She was so obsessed with getting back to her life on the farm that she missed out on enjoying some of the incredible opportunities Oz had to offer. She never even TRIED to ride the Horse of a Different Color! And, honestly, when we dwell on the past, we're potentially missing out on magic horses too. When I first got diagnosed with depression, I kept saying, "I miss the old me," instead of appreciating the f*cking cool person I was becoming.

Are there things about the past you dwell on? List them here!

_____

_____

_____

_____

_____

_____

How did these things change your life?

_____

_____

_____

_____

_____

_____

**An affirmation about letting go of the past:** I accept that I can't change my past, but I can change my future.

# WHERE DOES THE TIME GO?

Let's say you rip your T-shirt. Instead of sewing it up or putting on a new shirt, you opt to put on a sweatshirt over it. But then when that sweatshirt inevitably gets spaghetti sauce all over it, you put on a jacket over that and then a gigantic feather boa over that, and the cycle continues. Like, yeah, you can't see the ripped T-shirt, but the more layers you put on, the more likely you are to overheat. This has been a metaphor for

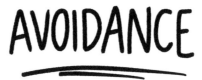

AVOIDANCE

Here's the thing about distractions (and jackets, for that matter): they aren't inherently harmful. It's totally okay and arguably necessary to zone out watching *The Holiday* every once in a while. What we need to keep an eye out for are the times you didn't even plan on zonking out while scrolling through TikTok; it just happened, and now it's suddenly 2 a.m., which sucks because you have to get up at

7 a.m. for work, and oh my freaking god, how did this happen AGAIN?! As we've established, life already sucks enough without the addition of time lost to mindless distractions.

For this exercise, don't worry about *why* you're avoiding stuff. Label all the distraction jackets with what you do when you want to avoid a task (or person or thought or emotion).

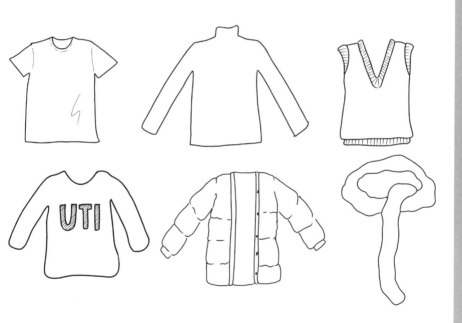

# POMO:
## PAIN OF MISSING OUT

Anxiety and depression can cause two kinds of pain: the pain of feeling anxious and/or depressed (duh), and the lesser-known pain of missing out on the things we're avoiding. POMO is a huge pain in the @ss!

**TMI Time:** In elementary school, I used to purposely miss field trips because I had anxiety about people throwing up on me. I memorized strep symptoms so I could convincingly act sick and would experience a brief moment of intoxicating relief when my mom agreed to let me stay home. But then, for the next twenty-four hours, I sat in bed wondering what my friends were doing. The next day at school, I'd hear about Mike C. leading a hilarious rendition of the *Flintstones* theme song on the bus or the surprise stop at a goat-petting zoo and be filled with regret. No one threw up, even a little bit. I'd missed out on a cool day just because I was scared of what *might* happen. It was a lose-lose situation. Nowadays, when I do things even when I'm scared, I do it for fourth-grade me. I know she'd be proud.

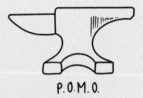

P.O.M.O.

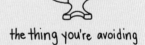

the thing you're avoiding

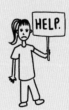

HELP.

Use the columns below to describe some times you've been hit by POMO:

| WORRY | WHAT I MISSED BECAUSE OF THE WORRY |
|---|---|
|  |  |
|  |  |
|  |  |
|  |  |
|  |  |
|  |  |
|  |  |
|  |  |
|  |  |
|  |  |
|  |  |
|  |  |
|  |  |

# OUR SOUL BATTERY

Inside each of us hums a powerful soul battery. It's where we find energy for loving, working, and petting (dogs). And just like a regular old phone battery, we need to make sure it stays charged. This means plugging into things that fill us with energy and regulating things that drain us.

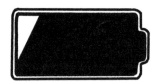

Think about how you feel when your soul battery is *full*. How is your mood, your sleep, and the way you interact with others?

And how do you feel when your soul battery is *depleted*? Don't forget to think about your self-talk, your energy, and your willingness to go with the flow.

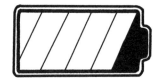

Let's figure out how certain activities affect your soul battery. Put a positive (+) or negative (—) sign next to each item to show what's filling you and what's draining you.

[ ] Responding to emails

[ ] Cooking dinner

[ ] Cleaning your room

[ ] Cleaning your work space

[ ] Exercising

[ ] Listening to music

[ ] Picking up an unexpected phone call

[ ] Talking to your family on the phone

[ ] Making a doctor's appointment

[ ] Doing accounting work, like taxes
or bookkeeping

[ ] Reading books

[ ] Going to a concert

[ ] Watching a movie

[ ] Rewatching a movie you liked when
you were younger

[ ] Watching a new TV show

[ ]   Watching reruns of your favorite old TV show

[ ]   Binge-watching a TV show

[ ]   Sleeping in

[ ]   Waking up early

[ ]   Going to bed late

[ ]   Going to bed early

[ ]   Showering in the morning

[ ]   Showering at night

[ ]   Putting on makeup

[ ]   Styling your hair

[ ]   Making your bed

[ ]   Perusing dating apps

[ ]   Having sex

[ ]   Drinking water

[ ]   Journaling

[ ]   Painting

[ ]   Freewriting (with writing prompts)

[ ]     Looking at social media

[ ]     Posting on social media

[ ]     Responding to texts from close friends

[ ]     Swapping memes with friends

[ ]     Having alone time

[ ]     Spending time with one other person

[ ]     Spending time with two people or more

[ ]     Going for a walk

[ ]     Spending time in nature

[ ]     Trying a new art form

[ ]     Doing art you feel very comfortable with

[ ]     Editing your work

[ ]     Filming yourself

[ ]     Watching tutorials to learn new skills

[ ]     Making new friends

[ ]     Talking to strangers

[ ]     Small talk

[ ]  Coffee

[ ]  Tea

[ ]  Finding parking

[ ]  Going to a new place

[ ]  Taking a big trip

[ ]  Typing

[ ]  Writing with a pen

[ ]  Working on art for fun

[ ]  Working on art to sell

[ ]  Working on art to give as a gift

[ ]  Gardening

[ ]  Yard work

[ ]  Meal prepping

[ ]  Grocery shopping

[ ]  Clothes shopping

[ ]  Public speaking

[ ]  Taking a nap in the middle of the day

[ ]  Procrastination

[ ]  Brainstorming

[ ]  Outlining

[ ]  Planning ahead

[ ]  _____

[ ]  _____

[ ]  _____

[ ]  _____

[ ]  _____

**Hot Tip:** Be honest with yourself and ignore what you think "should be" a positive or negative. Sometimes a positive activity has a negative impact on your battery. An example is cleaning your room. For some people, the act of cleaning is suuuuch a positive that it gives them much creative energy. For me, that's a huge drain. Having a clean space is awesome, so I need to do it, but then I need to balance it out with voltage elsewhere. (Can you tell I know jack sh*t about electricity? I don't know what a volt is. Anyway. Just keep that in mind—everyone is different, so no one's list will look the same.)

# DOWN THE DRAIN

Let's take a closer look at what's draining your soul battery. Pick five things you marked as negative (—) in the last exercise. Next to each one, write how much time that activity takes from your day.

Now look at your list and cross out any of the activities you could delegate. Put an X next to any that you could spend less time doing. Circle the ones that suck but are just part of life. Congratulations! You're already on your way to accepting that there will *always* be stupid life stuff sucking energy out of us. Some of it is out of our control, and some of it is necessary to make room for our dream life.

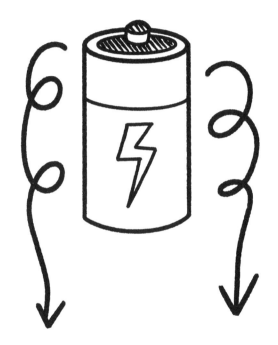

# TESTING POSITIVE

Okay, enough with all that negative crap. What supercharges your soul battery?! Choose five positive things from the last exercise and write them here:

1. _____

2. _____

3. _____

4. _____

5. _____

Write down how much time each of these things takes. You miiiight be surprised that something like "meal prepping" (—) can take the length of a *RuPaul's Drag Race* episode (+). How can you include more of that good sh*t into your daily (or at least weekly) life? Are there any positive activities you could do during negative ones, like listening to your favorite music while doing laundry or taking dance breaks during boring work calls? (Camera off, unless you're a daredevil.)

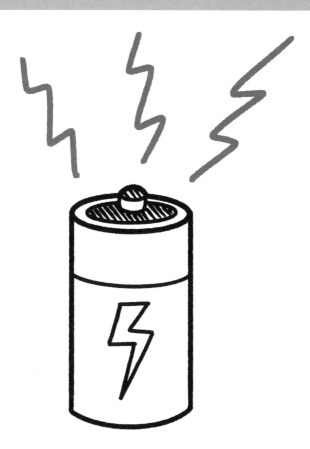

**An affirmation for keeping your battery charged:** I accept that I have to do things that drain my soul battery, because being a grown-up sucks a lot of the time. But sometimes I can balance the suckage by fitting recharging activities into my life, and for that I am grateful.

# GET YOUR SH*T STRAIGHT

I'd like to introduce you to my pal, Eisenhower. As in Dwight D. Eisenhower, thirty-fourth president of the United States . . . obvs. He came up with a genius way of organizing daily tasks based on their urgency and importance, which he used for, like, presidential sh*t. Later, author Stephen R. Covey created this chart so us regular folks could apply Dwight's philosophy to our own less presidential (but still important) lives. It's a surefire way to avoid that dreaded late-afternoon feeling of "What did I even do today?" Go on, give it a whirl! Fill this in using one of your recent to-do lists.

# Eisenhower's Matrix
**(Not to Be Confused with Keanu Reeves' _Matrix_)**

**IMPORTANT & URGENT**

**NOT IMPORTANT & URGENT**

**IMPORTANT & NOT URGENT**

**NOT IMPORTANT & NOT URGENT**

# ARE YOU SUUUURE?

Let's take a moment to examine what you wrote in the preceding exercise. Ask yourself: Are these tasks urgent and important to me, or to someone else? Is there actually a ticking clock, or is the urgency coming from somewhere else? Our definitions of "urgent" and "important" have been warped, especially thanks to the internet and the barrage of notifications we face from the moment we wake up to the moment we lay our beautiful little heads to sleep. The first time I filled out the Eisenhower Matrix, I put "responding to work emails" and "posting to Instagram" in the Important & Urgent category while "hanging out with friends" and "exercising" ended up in the Not Important & Not Urgent category. This reflected my lifestyle back at me: I valued making myself available to coworkers and strangers on the internet more than I valued my own emotional and physical health. So, with that in mind, let's take another go at this:

**An Important but Not Urgent Affirmation:** I accept that the immediacy of internet communication and the constant pressure to be a ridiculously productive member of society causes my brain's Urgency Radar to go batsh*t. Luckily, I can check in on what is actually urgent and what just *feels* urgent.

# REDO

**IMPORTANT & URGENT**

**NOT IMPORTANT & URGENT**

**IMPORTANT & NOT URGENT**

**NOT IMPORTANT & NOT URGENT**

# STARTING FROM THE BOTTOM

Here's another cool thing about Eisenhower's Matrix: it gives us the opportunity to delegate. Anything on the unimportant bottom half might be sucking time away from the important stuff on the top half. And, speaking from experience, when unimportant tasks get overwhelming and drain our soul battery, anxiety has a way of creeping in big-time.

Who are some people you can ask for help with
Eisenhower's bottom?

_____

_____

_____

_____

_____

_____

_____

_____

_____

_____

_____

_____

**Hot Tip:** Ask a pal to swap appointment-
making duties: they call and make yours, so
you call and make theirs. For some reason,
scheduling appointments for my friend is 1000
percent easier than scheduling them for myself.

# LET'S GET PHYSICAL

Bonus points if you use crayons or colored pencils or whatever the f*ck you accidentally bought the last time you were depressed in a craft store. What are some of the physical sensations you associate with these feelings?

_____

_____

_____

_____

_____

_____

_____

LABEL WHERE YOU FEEL THESE
EMOTIONS IN YOUR BODY:

**FEAR**

**ANGER**

**SADNESS**

**ANXIETY**

**JEALOUSY**

You know the drill. What are some of the physical sensations you associate with these feelings?

_____

_____

_____

_____

_____

_____

_____

_____

LABEL WHERE YOU FEEL THESE
EMOTIONS IN YOUR BODY:

**JOY**
**HOPEFULNESS**
**AMUSEMENT**
**EXCITEMENT**
**PEACE**

# IS THIS FOREVER?

Time to let that sh*t GO. Think back to some times when you've felt overwhelmed by negative emotions. What coping mechanisms helped you the most? Jot them down here. Don't worry about *how* or *why* they worked! That's for the scientists to worry about.

# DON'T YOU KNOW THAT YOU'RE TOXIC?

Positivity becomes toxic when it implies that the only correct response to sadness is happiness and that trouble should always be met with cheerful resistance. That's bullsh*t. When life gets cloudy, you don't have to find a silver lining. Instead, accept that there's a f*cking thunderstorm happening and get out of the pool for a while! You are entitled to feel *all* your emotions, in *all* their complexity.

Let's brainstorm (pun intended) other emotions that are just as powerful—and meaningful—as happiness. For the record, being hungry doesn't count as an emotion, but *hangry* absolutely does.

_____

_____

_____

_____

_____

_____

_____

_____

_____

_____

_____

_____

_____

_____

_____

_____

_____

_____

_____

_____

_____

**An affirmation for emotional range:** I'm so much more than just happy or sad. I contain f*cking multitudes.

# MAYBE IT'S JUST
# WHO YOU ARE

~~~~~~~~~~~~~~~~~~~~~~~~~~~~~~~~

You know those people who just love adrenaline? They're in line for the most extreme roller coaster or buying tickets for the haunted house or asking to watch a mega-gruesome horror film at a sleepover. I have a confession: I'm not that person. And I'll never be that person. Accepting that I'm a sensitive wittle scaredy-cat who prefers *Shrek* to *Kill Bill* has changed my life for the better. It opened doors for me to also accept that I'm NOT a morning person, I'm DEFINITELY a cat person, and skipping lunch makes me extremely grumpy. Fill in some of these blanks to start your journey of accepting who you are RIGHT NOW:

**I accept that I will never be the kind of person who**

_____

_____

_____.

**And while we're on the topic, I get upset by**

_____

_____

_____,

**and I'm okay with that.**

**Someday, I might be able to**

_____

_____

_____,

**but I accept it will be difficult because**

_____

_____

_____.

**It might not be everyone's cup of frickin' tea, but I love**

_____

_____

_____.

**It makes me happy, OKAY? Maybe that's just who I am.**

# TAKE A DUMP . . .
# A WORRY DUMP

Take a deep breath, unclench your cheeks, and grab hold of something sturdy. We're taking a dump. A worry dump! Like the worst bouts of gas, worries can hurt your tummy unless you let them rip.

Use this page to write down every single worry bouncing around that creative little brain of yours.

Feel better?

# PART TWO

# Jealousy Is a Sickness

## (Get Well Soon, B*tch!)

*In which we turn jealousy into inspiration.*
*cue angels singing*

# "COMPARISON IS THE QUEEF OF JOY"

## —THEODORE ROOSEVELT, MAYBE

What if I told you jealousy isn't a bad emotion? Sure, it can certainly *feel* bad, but deep down, jealousy is giving you not-so-subtle hints about what you want in life. The next few exercises can help illuminate some of those dreams and desires so you can shut that green-eyed monster up. First, you need to identify who makes you feel jealous in different areas of your life. Don't be afraid to get radically honest here. They aren't going to see this workbook, and I am a very good secret keeper. So, who makes you jealous . . .

- In real life?
- On the internet?
- From childhood?
- From when you were a teen?
- At the gym?
- In magazines?
- In movies?
- In relationships?
- Inside your own brain?

**FOR EXAMPLE:** In real life, I'm jealous of anyone performing in a musical. On the internet, I'm jealous of people who regularly get their hair dyed outrageous colors. When I was a kid, I was jealous of the girl who could run a five-minute mile in PE. I won't name names, but I think you know who you are.

# DON'T BE A J-HOLE

Take a li'l looksie at that list you just made. Now, write down WHY you're jealous of these people. Was it because they were bragging about a new job? Posting a photo wherein their kids were wearing eerily clean white overalls? Something about them triggered your brain to be rude, as in "*They* have their life together. Which means YOU DON'T." Please share with the class:

> **TMI Time:** Personally, every time I see someone even close to my age buy a house, as in OWN property, as in become a HOMEOWNER . . . I get hit by a rage bus. Have all the babies and weddings you want, but buy a house and my head bursts into flames. (No offense to all my friends who've bought houses. I can be very happy for you and sad for myself at the same time.)

**WHO?**

**WHY?**

# PENCIL ME OUT

Choose one of those people from your jealousy list and imagine a REALISTIC day in their life. What does it look like?

**Morning:**

_____

_____

_____

_____

_____

_____

_____

_____

_____

_____

**Afternoon:**

_____

_____

_____

_____

_____

_____

_____

_____

_____

**Evening:**

_____

_____

_____

_____

_____

_____

_____

_____

_____

_____

**LOOK AT WHAT YOU WROTE.** Are you *sure* you imagined a REALISTIC day? A day that includes waking up at 5 a.m. to smile on a talk show, violently explosive diapers, wearing makeup to the gym? Try to imagine some real responsibilities, problems, and worries that your jealousy object has to deal with. When you're sure you've added some reasonably accurate IRL unpleasantness, go ahead and cross out all the things that you are glad *you* don't have to deal with.

**THEN ASK YOURSELF:** Do you truly think living this day of their life is any easier than living a normal day of your life? Jot down why.

# WHY DO I EVEN CARE?

**POP QUIZ!** Let's keep dissecting your feelings of envy. These questions should help you zero in on the core of what is making you feel less than.

**Do you feel jealous of other people because they have more money than you, or is it actually:**

**A**   How they make their money
**B**   The lifestyle they can afford with their money
**C**   Where they travel, thanks to their money
**D**   No, it's really the money.

**Do you feel jealous of that person's wedding, or is it actually:**

**A**   That it seems they've found their soulmate
**B**   The attention that they're getting
**C**   Their gigantic diamond ring
**D**   No, it's really the wedding

Do you feel jealous of other people's kids, or is it actually:

**A** The amount of time spent *away* from the kids
**B** How well behaved the kids seem
**C** How much money they spend on the kids' designer clothes
**D** No, it's really the kids

Do you feel jealous of that person's toned ass, or is it actually:

**A** The consistent time they set aside to do something for themselves
**B** Their confidence
**C** How many "likes" they get on their post
**D** No, it's really the ass

Do you feel jealous of that person's new house, or is it actually:

**A** The security of owning a home
**B** The way they seemed to have their life "together"
**C** That they have money for an outrageous house
**D** No, it's really the house

**If you answered mostly a's:** You might be less jealous of people's stuff and more jealous of how they're spending their time. Ask yourself: What is actually worth your time? What do you really want your days to look like?

**If you answered mostly b's:** This is VERY NORMAL, but you might actually be jealous of how other people's lives *seem*, rather than how their lives actually *are*. Being "put together"—whether it's broadcasting confidence at the gym or kids being polite on the playground—is almost always superficial. Odds are the people that make you jealous are fakin' it till they're makin' it, just like the rest of us.

**If you answered mostly c's:** You could be focusing on monetary value instead of actual value. Yes, the diamond ring is 6 carats and the toddler's pants are from Anthropologie, but that doesn't give them emotional, intellectual, or spiritual value. Try looking past the numbers and finding a new, less math-oriented definition of success.

**If you answered all d's:** It sounds like you are in tune with what you want. Go forth and continue your quest to get the money/wedding/ass/house of your dreams.

Are your feelings of jealousy surface-level, or are they the underbelly of an iceberg? How deep do these feelings go? Using the answers to this quiz, you can find ways to replace the time you spend being jealous with small goals that are in line with the actual thing you're jealous of. For instance, if you experience jealousy looking at an Instagrammer's taut booty pic, you can spin that green into gold by setting some time aside to work out. Just go for a walk! Now, look: you have a taut booty too, just in a different way. Spend time on your health, start a vacation savings fund, hire a babysitter, rob a bank, commit tax fraud—whatever! *Doing* something will put you back in control. And you can flip jealousy the bird.

# EVERYBODY POOPS

~~~~~~~~~~~~~~~~~~~~~~~~~~~~~

The rumors are true. Almost everybody poops in one way or another. All the people you included on your jealousy list? They've probably pooped. In a toilet, if they're lucky!

What other less-than-glam things do you and the people from your jealousy list have in common? No detail is too small! List them all here:

# YOUR PERFECT DAY

Imagine your most perfect day. You can dredge up a good memory or dream up a perfect day in the future. Not to be a party pooper, but try to stay *somewhat* grounded in reality. Although, if you insist on bending the rules of time, space, and bank account, make two lists: a realistic one and an aspirational one! Why the hell not?

**Perfect Morning:**

_____

_____

_____

_____

_____

_____

_____

_____

_____

_____

_____

_____

_____

_____

_____

_____

_____

_____

_____

**Perfect Afternoon:**

**Perfect Evening:**

_____

_____

_____

_____

_____

_____

_____

_____

_____

_____

_____

_____

_____

_____

_____

_____

_____

_____

_____

_____

# HONEY, I SHRUNK MY SCHEDULE

Full disclosure: I haven't *seen* what you consider a perfect day, but I am going to guess that it's not suuuuper attainable. Because if it were, we'd all just be living out our perfect days all the time and society as we know it would crumble.

But what if we try to create tiny, perfect *moments* as often as possible? Let's put aspects of your perfect day under a shrink ray. For instance, my perfect day involves waking up in Paris to the smell of my first cup of gorgeous, European espresso handcrafted by my sexy manservant, Jean-Pierre. I don't live in France and unless you tell A LOT of your friends to buy this book, I can't afford a manservant, but I do live in a time in history when I can order literally anything on the internet. *Et voilà!* I don't have to wait until I live in France or run a household staff to enjoy espresso first thing in the morning. I can find a perfect moment of espresso as soon as my espresso-making kit comes in the mail.

Your turn:

# Perfect Day

VERY REAL
SHRINK RAY

# Perfect Moment

# Perfect Day

# Perfect Moment

# Perfect Day

# Perfect Moment

_____

_____

_____

_____

_____

_____

_____

_____

_____

_____

_____

_____

_____

_____

_____

_____

_____

_____

# USING JEALOUSY AS ROCKET FUEL

It's easier to go after what we want when we actually know what we want. Review the last few exercises and fill in this very scientific Venn diagram:

*Huge shout-out to Venn—whoever you are!

YOUR PERFECT DAY

JEALOUSY

ROCKET
FUEL

# HITTING THE G-SPOT

Have you ever said this: "I shouldn't feel sad because I am SO lucky and there are MILLIONS of people who have it WORSE than I do, which is why I am a pee-pee poo-poo ungrateful little slob"? So, you're telling me that you compare yourself to people who (appear to) have it way better than you AND also to people who (appear to) have it way worse than you?! Oh, baby—no. Give yourself a break. Your brain can find a surprising amount of peace just by focusing on the good stuff here and now. So let's give a shout-out to the things you're grateful for. Remember, being grateful doesn't necessarily mean *happy* or *thankful*. Being grateful can simply mean *noticing* and *appreciating*.

Try this exercise: notice three good things.

# Three things right in front of you:

1. _____
2. _____
3. _____

# Three people in your life:

1. _____
2. _____
3. _____

# Three aspects of who you are as a person:

1. _____
2. _____
3. _____

# Three places you've visited:

1. _____
2. _____
3. _____

# Three cool (or uncool, f*ck it!) things you've learned in your life:

1. _____
2. _____
3. _____

# Three things you're looking forward to in the near future:

1. 
2. 
3. 

# Three things you're looking forward to in the distant future:

1. 
2. 
3.

# GIVE A F*CKING COMPLIMENT

If gratitude gives you the ick, no problem. Here's another exercise that can provide similar benefits!

# Pick five objects in the room and compliment the sh*t out of them.

1. 
2. 
3. 
4. 
5. 

# Think of three people you see sometimes and compliment the sh*t out of THEM!

1. 
2. 
3. 

Compliment yourself. Do it. I triple-dog-dare you.

# MEMO: TAKE THE F*CKING COMPLIMENT

Have you ever heard: "Talk to yourself like you'd talk to your best friend"? It's a beautiful sentiment, but personally it's never worked for me. However, I have found some success talking to myself like I'm my own overeager coworker, sending a very professional memo. I think it's because I would never put "you're a big dumb idiot" in a work email. Try writing yourself a very professional memo about accepting the compliments you've received from other people. I'll help you get started . . .

```
□□□
```

------------------------------------------

Subject: Re: Accepting Compliments

Hey!

Wanted to pass on some of the amazing
feedback you've received. Here are
some compliments people have given
you: (list compliments here). Really
great work. Can we circle back on how
you'll take these compliments as truth
instead of discrediting them?

Let me know if you have any questions!

All the best,

------------------------------------------

# YOU DESERVE
# A (P)RAISE

A lot of motivational posters and self-help Instagram accounts will tell you that NO ONE else's opinion matters. The only person you can trust is YOURSELF, so F*CK everyone. Who cares what they think?! Yeah, okay. I'll just never care what anyone else thinks ever again. Easy-peasy. I hope it's obvious that I'm being sarcastic. As the great Barbra Streisand sings, "People who need people are the luckiest people in the world." Who are some people whose opinions matter to you? Is it possible to ask them for positive feedback on a regular basis? How?

_____

_____

_____

_____

_____

_____

_____

_____

_____

_____

_____

_____

_____

_____

_____

_____

_____

_____

**TMI Time:** I find it helpful to call friends and straight-up ask them to say they are proud of me. Sometimes you can't get what you want unless you ask for it.

# THROW YOUR PHONE INTO THE OCEAN

Great news! Society (yes, all of society, every single person on the planet) just hopped on a call and decided we don't need phones anymore. No more scrolling, no more swiping, no more 11 p.m. email notifications. You'll have to get your news from the Pony Express and only feel jealous of your next-door neighbors instead of every single fashion blogger and person you went to middle school with.

Use this space to come up with as many creative ways to get rid of your phone as possible. Personally, I want to melt mine down and wear it as sparkly jewelry.

_____

_____

_____

_____

_____

_____

_____

_____

_____

Okay, so here's the bad news: society didn't really hop on a call and decide we don't need phones anymore. They're f*cking here to stay, _apparently_, so go fish your phone out of the ocean and use this page to brainstorm some more realistic ways you can limit how much time you spend cooking those beautiful eyes on a phone screen.

_____

_____

_____

_____

# WORRY DUMP:

## THE SEQUEL

~~~~~~~~~~~~~~~~~~~~~~~~~~~~~~~~

Pretend your brain is a sponge, soaked with worries.
Ring. It. Out.

**An affirmation for recovering doom-scrollers:**
I accept that I need my phone to be a
productive member of society, but I have power
over how much time I spend looking at it.

# PART THREE

# F*cking Deal with It!

Accept that sometimes things just suck
(and sometimes they also don't suck).

Our painful experiences aren't a liability—they're a gift.
They give us perspective and meaning, an opportunity to
find our unique purpose and our strength.

**—DR. EDITH EVA EGER**

# YOUR BRAIN IS AN IDIOT (NO OFFENSE)

In order to truly DEAL WITH OUR THOUGHTS, we need to be able to look *at* them, rather than *through* them. When we look *through* our thoughts, we're basically letting our thoughts color our whole perception. Which is how we end up saying things like "This has been the WORST day," and "I'll NEVER learn how to play 'Jingle Bells' on electric guitar." I mean, yeah. With that attitude, you definitely won't. In the left column, I'm going to share some thoughts that, if we look *through* them rather than *at* them, look like facts. In the right column, I'll present a more ACT-fueled way of looking *at* each thought.

| | |
|---|---|
| **I suck at martial arts.** | I currently suck at martial arts. But if I keep practicing, who knows how great I'll get! |
| **This is the worst week of my life.** | A lot of stuff that caused me to feel bad happened this week. Good thing there's next week. |
| **I made another mistake at work. My boss is going to fire me.** | Drats! I'm a human being who made an error, just as I was put on this earth to do. I could ruminate on the negative thoughts I'm noticing, but judging from past experiences that could lead to me feeling way worse. Instead, I'll reach out to the person whose LITERAL JOB is to support other people in their work environment. |
| **I'm a terrible partner. I don't deserve love.** | I'm experiencing a worry about my relationship. Better check in with my partner so I don't jump to any weird, devastating conclusions. |
| **If I can't break a board with my fists, I can't do anything.** | My accomplishments don't dictate my worth. I am so much more than my ability to break (or really hurt my hand on) a board. |

# OKAY, BUT WHAT IF YOUR BRAIN WAS A PUPPY?

It's hard to separate yourself from your brain! But maybe it would be easier if you imagined your brain as a puppy. (Or if you're not a dog fan, maybe imagine your brain as a hamster or a bearded dragon— whatever works!)

name me!

Name your puppy:

Describe your brain/puppy. What kind of fur does it have? Is it a loud, yappy puppy or a quiet no-barking pup? A sociable pooch or a shy pupster?

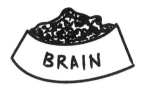

BRAIN

Aw, your puppy sounds so cute! Let's imagine your puppy takes a gigantic poop in your house. Well, that's gross. "I wish I hadn't fed you that expensive beef stew, little puppy," you might say. The puppy understands it did something wrong and is ashamed. You have a choice here. You could get super PO'd at the puppy, yell at it, and send it outside in the cold—making it (and yourself) more miserable.

Or you could observe that the puppy is separate from its super-gross poop. You still love your puppy, even if it made a mistake. You can politely ask your puppy to poop outside instead of on your beautiful beige sofa (wow, you have great taste!), but no matter where it happens, the puppy is going to poop. Hopefully, it's outside on a perfectly sunny day when you are prepared with a plethora of doggy poo bags. But, honestly, there will be days when you have to pick up your puppy's excrement late at night when it's hailing and −2 degrees. That might suck extra, but odds are it doesn't make you love your puppy any less. I mean, look at those ears!

**Doodle your puppy and its poop to
demonstrate that they are separate:**

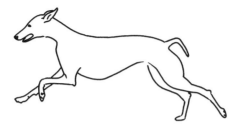

Luckily, in between the pooping and scooping, you and your puppy have a lot of fun. It chases squirrels and enjoys treats and cuddles with you on the couch. Watching your puppy interact with the world brings you more joy than you could've ever imagined. If you'd kicked your puppy out of the house when it took a doo-doo in the living room, you would've missed all of these adorable moments!

Okay, so get this: Your brain *is* like your puppy. It's going to have shitty thoughts. Because that's just what it does! It's a brain; it biologically cannot avoid negative emotions ALL THE TIME. If you get mad at your brain every time it metaphorically takes a poop in your living room, you AND your brain will be miserable. Be kind to your puppy. Be kind to your brain. And maybe invest in some quality carpet cleaner.

# YOUR PUPPY BRAIN, PART 2

If it's okay with you, I'd like to go even deeper with this puppy metaphor. I'm no psychic, but I bet a few of you read the last section about puppy doo-doo and went straight to "Well, I'll just train the puppy not to do that." In order for this metaphor to work, we gotta throw out the notion of puppy training. If, in real life, you lived with a puppy who regularly shat all over your 600 sq. ft. apartment, all your friends and I would encourage you to find a fancy puppy academy, or at the very least a wikiHow article on K9 obedience. But this is a metaphor and I'm sort of in charge. So no puppy training.

Imagine you and your puppy are on a walk and you trot past a mail delivery person. Your puppy goes bananas: growling, barking, pulling on its leash, teeth bared. It's terrifying! You release your puppy's leash so it can run straight to the poor postie's ankles and sink its tiny, razor-sharp teeth right into their leg. Fired up, you get down on all fours and bite the other leg. So what if your parents spent thousands of dollars on your braces? Your puppy's alerting you to danger, and you're throwing yourself into the fray. Which would

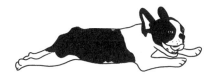

be, like, really dumb, right? No shame! We've all been there. Your brain is going to try to protect you from every perceived danger in the world, even the ones that are actually quite harmless, like the mail delivery person, or a fuzzy-wuzzy squirrel, or a public speaking opportunity. It's up to you, the brain owner, to decide how to respond. Anxiety and depression (heck, simply existing in this bonkers world) can cause us to forget we have this power. You're holding the leash. If your brain puppy starts losing its sh*t over whatever comes around the corner, you have the ability to hang on, take a second of rational evaluation, and decide not to attack a metaphorical random person on the street.

In real life, this could manifest in different, probably familiar ways. Oftentimes, we hear our brain puppy start barking and we don't even consider going on the attack. We usually run the other way, our scared puppy brain leading the way. If you're anything like me, you've missed many an event because the idea of meeting new people sets your brain puppy off. What are some things that have caused your brain puppy to lose its sh*t?

# BUT IF I'M NOT MY THOUGHTS, THEN WHO THE F*CK AM I?

Time for an art project! We've focused enough on your puppy; now it's time to focus on YOU. Use these pages to doodle all the different versions of you. Negative thoughts are not WHO you are; they are just something you have to deal with. You could be a student, a sibling, a friend, a volunteer—at the very least, you are definitely a literate person who cares enough about themselves to be filling out this workbook!

Now, tell me (or draw for me), who are you?

# I LIKE BIG BUTS

Now that we've established a healthy distance between us and our thoughts, let's turn our attention to memories. How many times have you been having a lovely day when— BOOM! a random upsetting memory shoves its way front and center in your mind? That kind of bullsh*t can mess with your head for weeks!

Because your brain is a sweet but very dumb puppy, you have to accept that memories are always going to be popping up. It's the equivalent of a puppy burying a disgusting tennis ball in the yard and digging it up every so often, just to make sure it's still disgusting. However, we have the power of BUTS. Negative memory comes up? Hit it with a BUT. Allow me to demonstrate. When I was twelve, I sang "America the Beautiful" at an assembly in front of my whole school. I couldn't hit the high note and my voice cracked, so I did what any unseasoned professional would do and started giggling so uncontrollably into the microphone that a teacher had to usher me off the stage. (Around this point in the memory, my heart rate speeds up and I'm tempted to swear off public appearances forever.) BUT thanks to that slipup, my threshold for embarrassment went sky-high. My period leaked through my pants during final exams? I got diarrhea in the fanciest grocery store in LA? Well, at least I'm not twelve, losing my mind in front of the whole school! See how powerful a BUT can be? For this exercise, I recommend starting small. Save the most traumatic memories for last—or, better yet, for therapy. And rest assured that "BUT I'm still here" is a perfectly valid answer.

| Memory | **BUT** | Reason I'm cooler because of it |
|---|---|---|
| | | |
| | | |
| | | |
| | | |
| | | |

**An affirmation of buts:** I accept that I can't change the past, but I can change my perception of it.

# WHAT EVEN IS ACCEPTANCE?

So I've been throwing around the word "accept" a lot in this book. It is, after all, a workbook based on *acceptance* and commitment therapy. Now seems like a good time to review what acceptance actually is, especially when it comes to mental health.

## ACCEPTING ≠ GIVING UP

If anything, it's the opposite. Acceptance is like buying a sandwich (trust me on this one). It's like buying a sandwich, sitting down at a sweet little table in the sun, opening the packaging, and realizing your sandwich is moldy. Gross. Giving up would mean tossing the sandwich into the garbage can and walking around hungry and feeling sorry for yourself the rest of the day. Pushing forward with no regard for your mental or physical health would mean eating the fuzzy blue sandwich anyway. And probably suffering even more later when you wake up at 2 a.m. with a belly full of regret. Both these choices lead to prolonged pain. Acceptance means acknowledging that your sandwich is moldy and understanding that you have the power to find yourself another meal. Sure, it's inconvenient in the moment, but that's better than spending the day hungry or the night puking your guts up. It's not the lunch you planned on, but it's the lunch you've been dealt. Seeking another option might cost you an extra few bucks, and it might take some extra time, but all of that is worth it. Because you deserve a lunch that isn't covered in spores.

And now, a quick survey:

**Did that moldy sandwich metaphor make any sense?**

☐ Yes
☐ No

**Do you feel that you could apply the moldy sandwich metaphor to your current life?**

☐ Yeah, it's causing me to rethink how I interact with the world.
☐ Please stop asking me questions.

**Would you consider thinking about that metaphor again in the future?**

☐ Sure.
☐ Seriously, I'm not really a metaphor person.

**On a scale of 1–10, how would you rate the metaphors in this workbook so far?**

☐ 10
☐ What do you want from me? A gold star?

Please draw a gold star right here:

Questions? Comments? Concerns?

_____

_____

_____

_____

_____

_____

_____

_____

_____

_____

# F*CK "TO-DO" LISTS!

We've spent our whole lives making to-DO lists and crossing things off. The more we cross off, however, it seems like the more we have to do. It never ends! But just *doing* things isn't what makes our lives valuable— it's the *being*. Being kind, being patient, being creative. Once we are *being* the way that we want, then we can DO literally anything. So, next we are going to make a to-BE list. Think about how you want to BE in your life.

**Your to-BE list:**

_____

_____

_____

_____

_____

_____

_____

_____

**"You are a human BEING, not a human DOING."**
—ONE OF MY PAST THERAPISTS

_____

_____

_____

_____

_____

_____

_____

_____

# SURPRISE!

Get excited, because between (hopefully) agreeing that you deserve better than a moldy-sandwich life and remembering who you want to BE, you've dipped your toe into the magical realm of the C in ACT: commitment. Commitment isn't simply promising that you'll do something. If that were the case, we would stick with regular ol' to-do lists and you could use this workbook as kindling. Commitment is twofold: the first part is unearthing your values, knowing how you want to exist in the world, a.k.a. your to-be list. Once you know HOW you want to be, you don't have to worry so much about what you DO. For example, if you put "be a good friend," you can BE a good friend right this very second. Think nice thoughts about your friends, give them a call, send them a meme. Look at you go! Living according to your values. Values can range from general stuff like "be kind," to more specific, like "be a present father figure." Meditating on your values can help you understand what you want. If you wrote "be a present father figure," this could be a not-so-subtle sign you want kids of your own in the future. The second part of commitment is the simplest and toughest part of all: the actual being. Allowing yourself to experience the world through your values instead of your thoughts. Remember, our brains are IDIOTS (and dumb puppies), so they might be confused by this bit, but the key is practice. Practice being how you want to be every day. It won't always go smoothly, but you'll be more fulfilled just by trying. That's a lot of information. Reflect on your values and commitment here:

## Lifestyle

_____
_____
_____
_____
_____

## Family

_____
_____
_____
_____

## Home

_____
_____
_____
_____

## Money

---

---

---

---

---

## Love

---

---

---

---

---

## Health

---

---

---

---

---

## Career

_____

_____

_____

_____

_____

_____

_____

## Other Stuff

_____

_____

_____

_____

_____

# WORRY DUMP III: THE WORRY DUMP STRIKES BACK

Squeeze every single worry out of that beautiful sponge of a mind.

Just for funsies: Revisit your first two worry dumps (page 46 and 88), and check how many of those worries are still plaguing you. Have any of them resolved? If there are worries that have withstood the test of time, can you ask someone wiser than you for a new perspective? Maybe you are still stuck in some harmful habits that only someone who is not you could see.

# PART FOUR

# The Best Is Yet to Come, Baby!

Identify your core values and commit to live by them.

I never look back, darling. It distracts from the now.

**—EDNA "E" MODE,** *The Incredibles*

# YOUR
# NEW YORK TIMES
# BESTSELLER

Congratulations! You've just published your tell-all memoir that outlines the story of your life so far. Let's decorate the cover together.

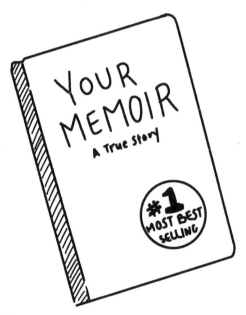

# FRONT COVER:

..................................................................

*What's the title?*

..................................................................

*The (Your Name Here) Story*

# BACK COVER:

..................................................................

..................................................................

..................................................................

..................................................................

..................................................................

..................................................................

..................................................................

Write a summary of the story of your life so far.

**"A book FULL of words."**
—CHRISTINA WOLFGRAM, author of *F*cking Deal With It*

**"Love their use of commas."**
—CHRISTINA'S MOM

**"Incredible spelling."**
—RANDOM TWITTER USER

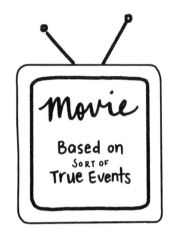

# LIGHTS, CAMERA, ACTION

Okay, wow. Your memoir has caused quite a stir, and now your story is being turned into a LIFETIME ORIGINAL MOVIE! There's one catch, though: The producers over there need you to spice up the story a bit. Don't add anything too out of the ordinary (we don't have much of a special F/X budget), but think about your to-be list, your goals, and what you'd want to do if you never felt scared of anything ever again. Write the script for the trailer of the Lifetime original movie based on your life. Remember, you're the main character, babycakes!

Now, someone get this star a freaking triple latte, extra hot! Chop-chop!

# CH-CH-CH-CHANGES

Examining the differences between what you wrote on your memoir cover and what you wrote for your Lifetime original movie trailer can be eye-opening. It might reveal some of the changes you want to make in your life that you may be pushing down under the iceberg or avoiding. What are some of the differences?

What are some of the characteristics of your Lifetime movie self you wish you possessed in your real life?

What does your Lifetime movie self have that you wish you, in real life, had too? For instance, does your dramatized self have a spouse or children or a pet? Do they live in a different city or have a different career? Where do they spend most of their time?

_____

_____

_____

_____

_____

_____

It's totally normal if you're noticing tension in your body or maybe upsetting memories bubbling up. Seeing the distance between who we are and who we wish we were can be, well, sucky. But remember, life is going to suck whether or not you make changes. So we might as well go for it!

_____

_____

_____

_____

_____

_____

# DEAR BRAIN, I FORGIVE YOU

At this point in the workbook, you've faced SO MUCH tough sh!t about being a human being on this god-forsaken planet. You've learned that our brains desperately cling to "normal," even if that means "miserable." But you are not your brain, my friend. You are the boss, the star of your own movie. You can embrace change, even when your brain is being a whiny puppy peeing everywhere at the thought of it. If regrets are coming up (why oh why did I sink all my money into that hot-pink Porsche!), notice them, but try choosing not to believe them. You've always done the best you could, and I'm so proud of you. The only way to move now is forward. But first, finish this letter:

Dear Brain,
I forgive you.

_____

_____

_____

_____

_____

_____

_____

_____

_____

_____

_____

_____

_____

_____

_____

_____

_____

_____

Love,

_____
(YOUR NAME HERE)

# SPARE SOME CHANGE

Drastic before-and-after photos, fad diets, and Anne Hathaway's transformation scene in *The Princess Diaries* have convinced us that the only life changes that work are BIG, UNCOMFORTABLE, SUPER-MEANINGFUL ONES. *Au contraire, mon ami!* *French laugh* Change can be any old random thing. It's the *choosing* change that really matters. Taking a slightly new route driving home, sleeping on the left side of the bed instead of the right, ordering vanilla instead of your usual chocolate—every time you choose to make even the smallest of changes, it positively affects your brain's ability to welcome more life- or hair-altering changes in the future. Think of it as weight lifting, and you're starting with the one-pound dumbbells: sure, they're light, but once you've lifted them for a few days in a row, you're stronger! So, what are some itty-bitty changes you can make this week?

_____

_____

_____

_____

_____

_____

_____

_____

_____

_____

_____

_____

_____

_____

_____

_____

**Hot Tip:** If you tell yourself you're going to make a li'l change, but days go by and you find yourself stalling, phone a friend. Actually, don't phone them. Are you trying to give them a panic attack? Text a friend. Tell them about the little change. You can explain the exercise, but you don't have to! Truth is, it can be easier to follow through on a promise to yourself if you've shared it with someone else.

# THE KINGDOM OF BOUNDARIES

Imagine you are the ruler of a kingdom, the Kingdom of

_____

(WHATEVER YOU WANT).

As royal head honcho, your job is to keep everything running smoothly while protecting everyone from ogres and trolls and whatever other dangerous sh*t lurks beyond

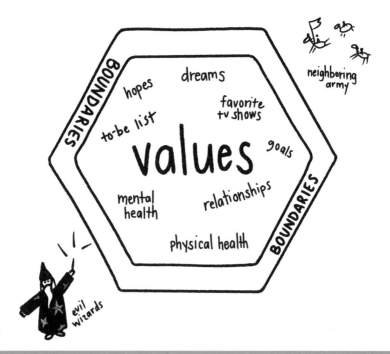

the castle walls. Think of those walls as boundaries between you and the world. A coworker who contacts you at 8 a.m. on a Saturday, an evil wizard seeking revenge, anything that disrupts your inner peace—put up a wall! And remember, walls can be varying heights; they can also have windows and doors. No wall is permanent. So check in on the castle walls every so often to ensure they are still working . . . and still necessary. What are some castle walls you want to build in your life?

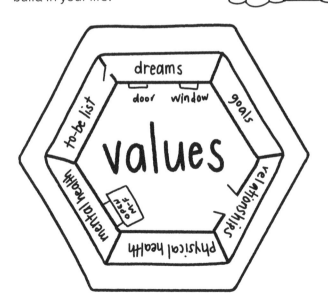

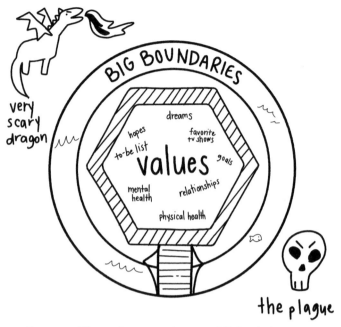

Because life sucks, as we've established, there may be far more menacing threats to your kingdom: fire-breathing dragons, the plague, or toxic people you need to cut out of your life, perhaps. For those forces of chaos, you build a moat. Moats are deep and offer more protection than walls. They last longer too. What would you want to keep out of your life with a moat?

There's one more kind of boundary to consider for the kingdom of your mind: the boundary between you and yourself. Maybe a more accurate name for this kind of boundary would be "promises"; if we can't keep promises to ourselves, how are we going to be able to enforce boundaries beyond the castle walls? Inside the castle, everyone has a job. Farmers

# YOUR TURN

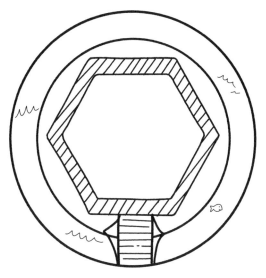

grow and harvest crops, blacksmiths use the hammer thing to shape horseshoes. Bakers bake and sewers sew and (cross your fingers) inventors invent indoor plumbing. But in order for everyone to be able to do their job, they need time and space, right? Maybe the baker loves to gossip, but the sewers get so distracted they don't sew enough pants for the kingdom. There should probably be a wall between the two. Like the main walls of the castle, these indoor rooms can have doors. They can be left open, or they can be locked. If people really want to get in, they can knock politely.

What kind of indoor walls do you want to build in your mind?

# X MARKS
# THE SPOT

*Whatever you're meant to do, do it now.*
*The conditions are always impossible.*

**—DORIS LESSING**

As my great-grandfather used to say, "Hot dog! What a ride! Where the hell are my cigarettes?!"

Congratulations on not only completing this workbook but also carving out the time and energy to examine what you want in life. The first step to getting what you want is *knowing* what you want, and I sincerely hope you've taken a big step toward understanding that part of yourself. Over the course of the last-however-many pages, you stared your fears in the face and decided to keep going anyway. You confronted how your interactions with the world around you affect your perceptions, you separated yourself from your thoughts, and you started to accept that we can't prevent shitty shit from happening.

Life will always be way better or way worse than anything we could ever imagine, so we might as well use our brainpower for other stuff. Like eating ice cream and kissing and upending the living room looking for the remote control. You've also endured a lot of metaphors. Like a LOT. But, do you have time for one last one? It's quick, I promise. I think it's normal to assume everything would be easier if we were born with a map of how our lives should go. It would tell us what the "right" decisions are and point us toward the direction of who we are "supposed" to be. But, my loves, we are the mapmakers. We can go anywhere, and that's scary—but exciting too. As we explore, guided by the light of our values, we get to discover that the treasure isn't at the end of the journey—it's scattered throughout.

None of it would be possible if you stayed second mate of your own ship. You're at the wheel now, so you can steer around the worry icebergs and stay the course you discovered during the past few exercises. Maybe, when you opened this book, you were floating. Now, you're the motherfucking captain of your life. Full speed ahead.

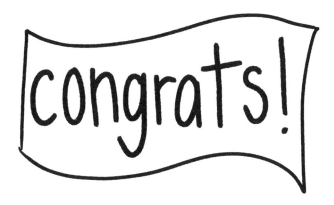

I contain F*cking multitudes

# Acknowledgments

This book would be but a smelly little brain fart without the work of Steven C. Hayes, the mastermind behind acceptance and commitment therapy. His workbooks explain gigantic ideas in such accessible, applicable ways that have helped me immensely in my day-to-day life. Thanks, Steven!

There aren't enough words in the English language to properly thank Sharyn Rosart for inviting me to develop this idea. Huge thanks to the whole beautiful team at Sasquatch Books: Jill, Tony, and Isabella especially.

I'd also like to acknowledge my family, friends who are family, Mister, West, Rosarita's Refried Beans, MPW, and anyone who has ever shared their mental health stories with me. Not to be dramatic, but hearing from you is the greatest honor of my life.

# Further Reading

BadBitchesHaveBadDaysToo.com

Megan Thee Stallion's amazing mental health website is a great place to start your search for a therapist or other resources. NAMI (National Association of Mental Illness) and Psychology Today also have databases that can connect you with mental health professionals.

*Get Out of Your Mind and Into Your Life: The New Acceptance and Commitment Therapy*
by Steven C. Hayes with Spencer Smith

Part workbook, part mind-blowing wisdom, this is the best next step for exploring ACT.

*Man's Search for Meaning*
by Viktor Frankl

Written by a psychiatrist who survived the Holocaust, this book proves that finding meaning, even in the darkest of circumstances, can keep us alive and keep us human.

*The Choice: Escaping the Past and Embracing the Possible*
by Edith Eger

Questioning humanity, identity, and how to live with trauma, this serves as a powerful companion to *Man's Search for Meaning*.

*The Artist's Way*
by Julia Cameron

This workbook will change your creative habits and open the artistic floodgates of your mind and heart.

*RuPaul: What's the Tee with Michelle Visage*

This podcast, especially the earliest episodes, contain so much love and wisdom. It's also where I learned about Saturn returns, which was obviously life changing.

# ABOUT THE AUTHOR

**CHRISTINA WOLFGRAM** is a sit-down comedian because she rarely stands up. Her musings on mental health, period cups, and waterproof mascara can be found all over the internet, most notably in the hit Facebook Watch show, *Christina Tried Her Best*. Christina is the proud owner of one whole master's in professional writing from USC and enjoys creating workshops that help people find their most authentic voice. Someday, Christina hopes to either win an exorbitant amount of money on a game show or get famous enough to get cast in a TV musical. In the meantime, she'll be updating *The Sob Blog* at cryingiscool.substack.com. Follow her on Instagram @itsthecwolf.

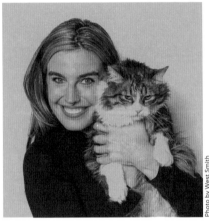